MEDITER

DIET

Mediterranean Diet: A Step-by-step Guide on How to Effortlessly Integrate a Healthy Diet Into Your Everyday Life

The Complete Mediterranean Diet Cookbook for Beginners

@ Victor Reed

Published By Adam Gilbin

@ Victor Reed

Mediterranean Diet: A Step-by-step Guide on How to Effortlessly Integrate a Healthy Diet Into Your Everyday Life

The Complete Mediterranean Diet Cookbook for Beginners

All Right RESERVED

ISBN 978-1-990053-70-2

TABLE OF CONTENTS

Pear Braised Pork

Ingredients:

- 1 bay leaf

- 1 thyme sprig

- 1 cup apple cider

- Salt and pepper to taste

- 3 pounds pork shoulder

- 4 pears, peeled and sliced

- 2 shallots, sliced

- 4 garlic cloves, minced

Directions:

1. Season the pork with salt and pepper.
2. Combine the pears, shallots, garlic, bay leaf, thyme and apple cider in a deep dish baking pan.
3. Place the pork over the pears then cover the pan with aluminum foil.

4. Cook in the preheated oven at 330F for 2 hours.
5. Serve the pork and the sauce fresh.

Balsamic Spring Onions Dip

Ingredients:

- 1 cup spring onions, chopped
- 1 teaspoon sweet paprika
- 1 cup veggie stock
- 3 red hot peppers, chopped
- A pinch of salt and black pepper
- 1 tablespoon balsamic vinegar

Directions:

1. In your instant pot, combine all the ingredients, put the lid on and cook on High for 8 minutes.
2. Release the pressure fast for 5 minutes, blend the mix using an immersion blender, divide into small bowls and serve.

Cream Cheese And Beef Spread

Ingredients:

- A pinch of salt and black pepper
- 1 teaspoon garlic powder
- 1 teaspoon rosemary, chopped
- 2 ounces cream cheese
- 1 cup cheddar cheese, shredded
- 1 yellow onion, chopped
- 1 tablespoon olive oil
- 1 pound beef, ground

Directions:

1. Set your instant pot on sauté mode, add the oil, heat it up, add the onion, beef and garlic powder, stir and brown for 5 minutes.
2. Add the rest of the ingredients, stir, put the lid on and cook on High for 15 minutes.

3. Release the pressure naturally for 10 minutes, stir the mix, divide into bowls and serve as a party spread.

Stuffed Chicken

Ingredients:

- 1 teaspoon hot paprika
- A pinch of salt and black pepper
- 1 cup tomato sauce
- 4 chicken breasts, skinless, boneless and butterflied
- 1 ounce spring onions, chopped
- 1 pound white mushrooms, sliced

Directions:

1. Flatten chicken breasts with a meat mallet and place them on a plate.
2. In a bowl, mix the spring onions with the mushrooms, paprika, salt and pepper and stir well.
3. Divide this on each chicken breast half, roll them and secure with a toothpick.

4. Add the tomato sauce in the instant pot, put the chicken rolls inside as well. put the lid on and cook on High for 30 minutes.
5. Release the pressure naturally for 10 minutes, arrange the stuffed chicken breasts on a platter and serve.

Cinnamon Baby Back Ribs Platter

Ingredients:

- 1 teaspoon onion powder

- 1 teaspoon cinnamon powder

- 1 teaspoon cumin seeds

- A pinch of cayenne pepper

- 1 cup tomato sauce

- 3 garlic cloves, minced

- 1 rack baby back ribs

- 2 teaspoons smoked paprika

- 2 teaspoon chili powder

- A pinch of salt and black pepper

- 1 teaspoon garlic powder

Directions:

1. In your instant pot, combine the baby back ribs with the rest of the ingredients, put the lid on and cook on High for 30 minutes.
2. Release the pressure naturally for 10 minutes, arrange the ribs on a platter and serve as an appetizer.

Buttery Carrot Sticks

Ingredients:

- 1 teaspoon rosemary, chopped
- A pinch of salt and black pepper
- 2 tablespoons olive oil
- 2 tablespoons ghee, melted
- 1 pound carrot, cut into sticks
- 4 garlic cloves, minced
- 1/2 cup chicken stock

Directions:

1. Set the instant pot on Sauté mode, add the oil and the ghee, heat them up, add the garlic and brown for 1 minute.
2. Add the rest of the ingredients, put the lid on and cook on High for 14 minutes.

3. Release the pressure naturally for 10 minutes, arrange the carrot sticks on a platter and serve.

Grilled Feta Spinach Salad

Ingredients:

- 1 tablespoon red wine vinegar

- 2 garlic cloves, minced

- 2 tablespoons extra virgin olive oil

- 8 oz. feta cheese, sliced

- 4 cups baby spinach

- 1/2 cup green olives, sliced

- 1/2 cup black olives, sliced

- 1 teaspoon capers, chopped

Directions:

1. Combine the baby spinach, green olives and black olives in a bowl.
2. For the Dressing:, mix the capers, vinegar and oil in a bowl.
3. Drizzle the Dressing: over the salad.

4. To finish it off, heat a grill pan over medium to high flame.
5. Place the feta cheese on the grill and cook on each side until browned.
6. Top the salad with the cheese and serve right away.

Chickpea Salad

Ingredients:

- 1 tablespoon lemon juice

- 1 can chickpeas, drained

- 1 cup chopped parsley

- 1 cup cherry tomatoes, quartered

- 4 oz. feta cheese, cubed

- 1 cup red grapes, halved

- Salt and pepper to taste

- 1/2 cup Greek yogurt

- 2 tablespoons extra virgin olive oil

Directions:

1. Combine the chickpeas, parsley, tomatoes, grapes and feta cheese in a salad bowl.
2. Add the rest of the Ingredients:and season with salt and pepper.
3. Serve the salad as fresh as possible.

Cajun Walnuts And Olives Bowls

Ingredients:

- 2 garlic cloves, minced
- 1 red chili pepper, chopped
- 1/2 cup veggie stock
- 2 tablespoon tomato puree
- 1 pound walnuts, chopped
- A pinch of salt and black pepper
- 1 and 2 cups black olives, pitted
- 1 tablespoon Cajun seasoning

Directions:

1. In your instant pot, combine the walnuts with the olives and the rest of the ingredients, put the lid on and cook on High 10 minutes.
2. Release the pressure fast for 5 minutes, divide the mix into small bowls and serve as an appetizer.

Kalua Pig

Ingredients:

- 1 cup water
- 1 tablespoon salt
- 1 cabbage, cut into wedges
- 6 lbs. pork roast, sliced
- 4 bacon slices
- 3 garlic cloves

Directions:

1. Set your instant pot to the sauté setting, and cook bacon slices for about 1-minute, cooking and browning all sides. Sprinkle salt on pork. Spread the salt on bacon evenly. Pour water into the instant pot and set to Manual mode.

2. Cover pot with lid and set on high with a cook time of 90-minutes. When the cook time is completed set the pot to the "Keep Warm" mode and release the pressure naturally for

10-minutes. Place the cooked pork in a bowl, taste the remaining liquid in the instant pot. Adjust seasoning as needed.

3. Now chop the cabbage and add it to the instant pot into the cooking liquid. Cover the pot once again and set on high with a cook time of 5-minutes.

4. When the cook time is completed, release pressure using quick-release. Serve the shredded pork with the cooked cabbage.

Pulled Apart Pork Carnitas

Ingredients:

- 1 teaspoon cumin
- 1 teaspoon garlic
- 1 teaspoon white pepper
- 2 teaspoons oregano
- 1 large onion, finely chopped
- 1/8 teaspoon cayenne pepper
- 1/8 teaspoon coriander
- 4 lbs. pork roast
- 2 tablespoons olive oil
- 1 head butter lettuce
- 2 grated carrots
- 2 limes, wedge cut
- Water
- 1 tablespoon salt

- 1 tablespoon cocoa

- 1 tablespoon red pepper flakes

Directions:

1. Add the "spice" Ingredients:in a bowl and mix them well.

2. Season the roast with the prepared mixture and chill the roast in your fridge overnight.

3. Set your instant pot to the sauté mode and add the olive oil and heat it.

4. Add the meat and brown it well.

5. Add water to the instant pot to submerge meat (about 1 cup).

6. Secure the lid of the pot in place, and set to Manual mode, on high with a cook time of 60-minutes.

7. When the cook time is completed, release the pressure naturally for 15-minutes.

8. Remove the meat from pot and shred the meat from bones.

9. Set your instant pot to sautė mode, simmer to reduce some of the liquid.

10. Add the shredded pork to a pan set over medium heat and stir-fry them until slightly browned.

11. Add some olive oil and spices.

12. Serve fried pork with the sauce from instant pot.

Pineapple Pork Chops

Ingredients:

- Balsamic glaze as required

- 6 pork chops, bone-in

- 1 cup cubed pineapple

- Olive oil as needed

- Seasoning of your choice for pork chops

Directions:

1. Season the pork chops. Set your instant pot onto the sautè mode.
2. Add the oil and heat it.
3. Add the chops to the pot and sautè them for a 5-minutes.
4. Remove the chops and place them onto a steamer rack for instant pot.
5. Glaze the pork chops and place the pineapple chunks on top of them.
6. Add a cup of water into the instant pot.

7. Secure the lid to pot and set to Manual mode, on high with a cook time of 25 minutes.

8. When the cook time is completed, release the pressure naturally for 10-minutes.

Apple Pork Tenderloins

Ingredients:

- 2 medium-sized green apples, sliced

- 3 lbs. boneless pork loin roast

- 2 tablespoons butter

- 1 large red onion, thinly sliced

- 1 teaspoon ground black pepper

- 1 teaspoon salt

- 1/2 cup chicken broth

- 2 bay leaves

- 4 thyme sprigs, fresh

Directions:

1. Set your instant pot to the sauté mode, add the butter and heat it.
2. Add the tenderloin pieces and cook them for 8-minutes.
3. Remove the cooked loins to a serving platter.

4. Place the red onion slices into the pot and sautè for 3-minutes.

5. Stir in the bay leaves, thyme, and apple slices.

6. Add broth along with pepper and salt, stir.

7. Add the loins back to the pot. Secure the pot lid and set on Manual mode on high with a cook time of 30-minutes.

8. When the cook time is completed, release the pressure naturally for 10-minutes.

9. Discard the bay leaves and transfer the pork to a cutting board and allow it to sit for 5-minutes.

10. Serve pork with sauce from pot.

Pork Shoulder Meal

Ingredients:

- 5 garlic cloves, minced

- 1 teaspoon cumin, ground

- 1 teaspoon salt

- Chopped cilantro, fresh for garnish

- 3 lbs. boneless pork shoulder,

- Cut into 2-inch cubes

- 1/2 cup orange juice

- 1/2 cup lime juice

Directions:

1. Add your lime juice, orange juice, cumin, garlic, and salt to your instant pot and stir to blend.

2. Place the pork into the instant pot and toss to mix.

3. Secure the lid to pot and set to Manual mode, on high with a cook time of 45-minutes.

4. When the cook time is completed, release the pressure naturally for 10-minutes.

5. Pre-heat your grill, using tongs take your pork out of the instant pot and place it on a baking sheet.

6. Set the instant pot to the sautė mode and cook for 10-minutes to allow liquid to reduce.

7. Pour the liquid into a heat-proof dish.

8. Broil the pork for 5-minutes or until crispy and serve with sauce, garnish with fresh cilantro.

Lamb & Feta Cocktail Meatballs

Ingredients:

- 1 cup breadcrumbs

- 2 tablespoons fresh parsley, finely chopped

- 1 tablespoon fresh mint, finely chopped

- 1 teaspoon kosher salt, plus more for sauce

- 1 tablespoon Worcestershire sauce

- 2 garlic cloves, crushed

- 2 lbs. lamb meat, ground

- 1 lb. feta cheese, crumbled

- 1 egg beaten

Directions:

1. In a large mixing bowl, add lamb, garlic, feta, egg, breadcrumbs, parsley, mint, salt, pepper and Worcestershire sauce.

2. Form mixture into 1-inch balls and place them in the freezer; allow them to harden for a few hours.

3. Add 1 cup water and steamer basket to your instant pot.

4. Lower the frozen meatballs onto the steamer basket.

5. Close and secure the lid to the pot.

6. Set on Manual mode, on high, with a cook time of 5-minutes.

7. When the cook time is completed, release the pressure using the quick-release.

8. Serve meatballs on a serving platter, serve with cocktail picks and one of your special sauces.

Instant Pot Lamb Shanks

Ingredients:

- 2 tablespoons ghee, divided

- Black pepper and salt as needed

- 3 cloves garlic, peeled, smashed

- 1 cup bone broth

- 1 teaspoon Fish Sauce

- 1 tablespoon vinegar

- 3 lbs. lamb shanks

- 1 tablespoon of tomato paste

- 1 large onion, roughly chopped

- 2 celery stalks, roughly chopped

- 2 carrots, medium-sized, roughly chopped

Directions:

1. Use salt and pepper to season lamb shanks.

2. Melt a teaspoon of ghee in your instant pot while in the sautė mode.

3. Add the shanks to pot.

4. Cook for 10-minutes, browning the shanks. Chop vegetables.

5. Remove the lamb from the pot.

6. Add veggies to pot and season them with some salt and pepper.

7. Add a tablespoon of ghee as well.

8. Once the vegetables are ready, pour garlic clove, tomato paste, into pot and stir.

9. Add in the shanks to veggie mix, along with tomatoes, bone broth, vinegar and fish sauce.

10. Close and secure lid, set to Manual mode on high, with a cook time of 45-minutes.

11. When the cook time is completed, release the pressure naturally for 10-minutes.

12. Serve lamb shanks and enjoy!

Inspiring Instant Pot Lamb Stew

Ingredients:

- 1 bay leaf

- 2 sprigs of rosemary

- 1 large yellow onion

- 3 large pieces of carrot

- 2 lbs. lamb stew meat cut up into 1-inch cubes

- 1 acorn squash

- 1/2 teaspoon salt

- 6 cloves garlic, sliced

Directions:

1. Peel the squash and deseed it, cube the squash.
2. Slice the carrots up into circles.
3. Peel the onion, slice in half and slice the halves into half moons.

4. Add all the Ingredients:into instant pot, close and secure pot lid.

5. Set pot to Manual mode, on high, with a cook time of 25-minutes.

6. When the cook time is completed, release the pressure naturally for 10-minutes.

7. Serve warm and enjoy!

Italian Style Baked Fish

Ingredients:

- 1/3 cup raisins

- 1 tbsp of lemon juice

- Black pepper to taste

- Parsley for garnishing

- Zest of one lemon

- 1.5 lb white fish fillet

- Mint for garnishing

- 1/3 cup olive oil

- 3 diced tomatoes

- 1.5 chopped red onion

- Ten chopped garlic cloves

- 1 tsp Spanish paprika

- 2 tsp coriander

- 1 tsp cumin

- 1.5 tbsp capers

- 1 tsp cayenne pepper

- Salt to taste

Directions:

1. Cook onions in heated olive oil in a saucepan for three minutes.

2. Stir in tomatoes, salt, capers, garlic, raisins, and spices and let them boil.

3. Reduce the flame to low and simmer for 15 minutes.

4. Rub fish with pepper and salt and set aside.

5. Transfer half of the cooked tomato mixture to the baking pan, followed by fish, lemon juice, zest, and leftover tomato mixture.

6. Bake in a preheated oven at 400 degrees for 18 minutes.

7. Sprinkle mint and parsley and serve.

Tzatziki Sauce And Dip

Ingredients:

- 1 tbsp minced dill

- 2 pinch of kosher salt

- 2 pinch of black pepper

- 1 halved cucumber

- 3/4 cup Yogurt

- 3 minced garlic cloves

- 2 tbsp red wine vinegar

Directions:

1. Place dried shredded cucumber in a bowl.
2. Mix garlic, vinegar, salt, yogurt, dill, and pepper in cucumber and mix well.
3. Cover the bowl and place it in the refrigerator. The Tzatziki sauce is ready.
4. Can store up to three days.

Pesto And Garlic Shrimp Bruschetta

Ingredients:

- 5 minced garlic cloves

- 3 oz pesto

- 2 oz capers

- 3 oz sun-dried tomatoes

- 1 oz feta cheese

- kosher salt to taste

- Glaze Balsamic for garnishing

- 8 oz shrimp

- Black pepper to taste

- 2 tbsp butter

- 4 tbsp olive oil

- 20 basil leaves

- 2 bread

Directions:

1. Sprinkle salt and pepper over shrimps in a bowl. Set aside for ten minutes.

2. Add olive oil and butter of about 2 tbsp each in the pan and cook for 2 minutes over medium flame.

3. Stir in garlic and sauté for one more minute.

4. Mix shrimps and cook for four minutes.

5. Remove from flame and let it set.

6. Slice the bread and place in a baking tray and drizzle oil and toast in the oven for five minutes.

7. Spread pesto sauce over each bread slice followed by sun-dried tomatoes, shrimp, caper, cheese, basil, and balsamic glaze and serve.

Pan-Seared Citrus Shrimp

Ingredients:

- 1 tbsp chopped red onion

- 2 pinch of red pepper flakes

- Kosher salt to taste

- Black pepper to taste

- 3 lb shrimp

- 2 wedge cut lemon

- 1 tbsp olive oil

- 6 tbsp cup lemon juice

- 1 cup of orange juice

- 2 sliced orange

- 6 minced garlic cloves

- 1 tbsp chopped parsley

Directions:

1. Mix parsley, pepper flakes, orange juice, oil, garlic, lemon juice, and onions in a bowl.

2. Transfer the onion mixture to skillet and cook over medium flame for eight minutes.

3. Add salt, pepper, and shrimps in a skillet and cook for five minutes or until shrimps are done.

4. Garnish with parsley and lemon slices and serve.

Cucumber And Tomato Salad

Ingredients:

- 2 tbsp olive oil

- Salt to taste

- 1 tbsp red wine vinegar

- Black pepper to taste

- 2 sliced English cucumber

- 1 sliced red onion

- 4 diced tomatoes

Directions:

1. In a large mixing bowl, mix all the Ingredients:and place in the refrigerator for 20 minutes.

2. Serve and enjoy it.

Citrus Avocado Dip

Ingredients:

- 1 cup chopped walnuts

- Black pepper to taste

- Cayenne as required

- Salt to taste

- 1 tbsp of lime juice

- 2 tsp sumac

- 1.75 oz shredded feta cheese

- 3 diced oranges

- 1 cup chopped onions

- 1 cup chopped mint

- 1 cup chopped cilantro

- Olive oil as required

- 3 sliced avocados

Directions:

1. In a bowl, combine all the Ingredients:and mix well.
2. Serve and enjoy it.

Roasted Tomatoes With Thyme And Feta

Ingredients:

- 3 tbsp olive oil

- Salt to taste

- 6 tbsp feta cheese

- 1 tsp dried thyme

- 16 oz cherry tomatoes

- Black pepper to taste

Directions:

1. In a baking tray, put tomatoes.
2. Pour olive oil and drizzle pepper, thyme leaves, and salt over tomatoes and mix well.
3. Bake in a preheated oven at 450 degrees for 15 minutes.
4. Drizzle cheese and broil for five minutes and serve when the cheese melts.

Greek Salad

Ingredients:

Dressing:

- 1/5 tbsp lemon juice

- 1.5 tsp minced garlic

- 1 tsp oregano

- 1.5 tbsp minced parsley

- 6 tbsp olive oil

- 2 tsp honey

- 1 tbsp red wine vinegar

- Salt to taste

Salad:

- 2 chopped green bell pepper

- 4 oz feta cheese

- 2 cup sliced Kalamata olives

- 2 chopped avocado

- 4 diced tomatoes

- 1 chopped onion

- 2 chopped English cucumber

Directions:

1. Whisk all the Ingredients:mentioned in the Dressing: list in a large mixing bowl. Set aside.

2. In another bowl, add all the Ingredients:of the salad and toss well.

3. Pour the Dressing:, toss well and serve.

Creamiest Hummus

Ingredients:

- 10 tbsp liquid from chickpeas can

- 2 tbsp lemon juice

- 1 tbsp olive oil

- 420 g chickpeas

- 1 tsp salt

- 8 tbsp tahini

Directions:

1. In a food processor, blend chickpeas, lemon juice, tahini, salt, and aquafaba to get smooth hummus.

2. Transfer the blended hummus to the bowl. Pour olive oil in the center of the hummus and serve.

Tahini Banana Shakes

Ingredients:

- 4 Medjool dates

- 3 sliced bananas

- 2 pinch of ground cinnamon

- 1/2 cup ice, crushed

- 2 cups almond milk

- 1/2 cup tahini

Directions:

1. Blend all the Ingredients:in the blender to obtain a creamy and smooth mixture.

2. Pour mixture in cups and serve after sprinkling cinnamon over the top.

Shakshuka

Ingredients:

- 1 tsp smoked paprika

- 1/2 tsp red pepper flakes

- 2 tbsp chopped cilantro for garnish

- 1 cup feta cheese

- 2 chopped yellow onion

- 28 oz fire-roasted tomatoes, crushed

- Crusty bread for serving

- 1 tsp ground cumin

- 2 tbsp olive oil

- 2 chopped red bell pepper

- 7 eggs

- 1/2 tsp salt

- 4 minced cloves garlic

- Ground black pepper to taste

- 2 tbsp tomato paste

Directions:

1. Heat oil in a skillet over medium flame and cook bell pepper, onions, and salt in it for six minutes with constant stirring.

2. After six minutes, stir in tomato paste, red pepper flakes, cumin, garlic, and paprika. Cook for another two minutes.

3. Add crushed tomatoes and cilantro to the onion mixture. Let it simmer.

4. Reduce the flame and simmer for five minutes.

5. Use salt and pepper to adjust the flavor.

6. Crack eggs in small well made at different areas using a spoon.

7. Pour tomato mixture over eggs to help them cook while staying intact.

8. Bake the skillet in a preheated oven at 375 degrees for 12 minutes.

9. Garnish with cilantro, flakes, and cheese and serve.

Simple Green Juice

Ingredients:

- 6 trimmed celery stalks

- 1 English cucumber

- 1 oz parsley

- 5 oz kale

- 1 tsp crushed ginger

- 2 apple

Directions:

1. Blend all the Ingredients:in the blender and pour into serving cups.

Greek Chicken Gyro Salad

Ingredients:

Chicken:

- 2 lb boneless chicken breasts

- 1 tsp ground black pepper

- 1 tbsp lemon juice

- 1 tsp Kosher salt

- 3 tsp dried oregano

- 2 tbsp olive oil

- 1 tbsp red wine vinegar

Salad:

- 1 cup diced tomatoes

- 1/2 cup diced red onions

- 1 cup crushed pita chips

- 1 cup diced English cucumber

- 6 cups lettuce

- 1 cup feta cheese diced

Tzatziki Sauce:

- 1 tbsp lemon juice

- 3/4 tsp ground black pepper

- 2 tsp dried dill weed

- 2 pinch of sugar

- 1 tbsp white wine vinegar

- 3/4 tsp Kosher salt

- 8 oz Greek yogurt

- 2 minced clove garlic

- 2/3 cup grated English cucumber

Directions:

1. Heat oil in a skillet and add chicken, salt, oregano, and black pepper.
2. Cook for five minutes over medium flame.
3. Reduce the flame to low and add lemon juice and vinegar and simmer for five minutes.
4. Continue cooking until the chicken is done.

5. Now, the chicken is ready and set aside.

6. Combine tomatoes, pita chips, chicken, lettuce, cucumber, and onions.

7. Mix and set aside. The salad is ready.

8. In another bowl, whisk yogurt, cucumber, garlic, lemon juice, vinegar, dill, salt, pepper, and sugar. Mix well. The sauce is ready.

9. Now, pour the sauce over the salad and serve with cooked chicken.

Tuscan Tuna And White Bean Salad

Ingredients:

- 1/4 cup sliced olives

- 1/2 cup diced cherry tomatoes

- 2 sliced red onion

- 1/2 lemon

- Kosher salt to taste

- 1/4 cup feta cheese

- Black pepper to taste

- 2 tbsp extra virgin olive oil

- 15 oz cannellini beans

- 4 cups spinach

- 5 oz white albacore

Directions:

1. Combine white beans, olives, lemon juice, arugula, onions, tuna, olive oil, and tomatoes in a mixing bowl.
2. Sprinkle pepper and salt and feta cheese and serve.

Outrageous Herbaceous Mediterranean Chickpea Salad

Ingredients:

- 3 tbsp lemon juice
- 3 minced cloves garlic
- 1/2 tsp kosher salt
- 2 chopped red bell pepper
- 1/2 tsp black pepper
- 1/2 cup chopped celery with leaves
- 30 oz chickpeas
- 1.5 cups chopped parsley
- 1/2 cup chopped onion
- 3 tbsp olive oil

Directions:

1. Combine bell pepper, onion, chickpeas, celery, and parsley in a mixing bowl.

2. In another bowl. Mix olive oil, garlic, salt, lemon juice, and pepper.
3. Pour olive oil mixture over chickpeas mixture and mix well and serve.

Tasty Vegetable And Fish Soup

Ingredients:

- 120 g haddock fillet

- 1 tbsp Worcestershire sauce

- 1 sprig of parsley

- 2 tablespoons of olive oil

- 1 pinch of salt and pepper

- 1 paprika

- 1 carrot

- 1 shallot

- 310 ml fish stock

Directions:

1. Firstly, half a pepper is pitted and cut into thin strips.

2. Next, the carrot and shallot are peeled and then finely diced.

3. Now a tablespoon of olive oil is heated in a saucepan.

4. In the heated oil, the peppers and the shallot and carrot cubes are lightly steamed for a minute.

5. Now the fish stock is added and everything is covered and left to simmer for five minutes.

6. Finally, the bite-sized fish fillets are added and everything is simmered again for five minutes.

7. The finished soup is now refined with a tablespoon of Worcestershire sauce, salt and pepper and sprinkled with parsley.

Trout Fillets With Zucchini Spaghetti

Ingredients:

- 2 tbsp pumpkin seed oil

- 2 dashes of lemon juice

- 1 teaspoon dried oregano

- 2 tablespoons of olive oil

- 1 pinch of salt and pepper

- 270 g trout fillets

- 2 zucchini

- 1 hot pepper

- 2 sprigs of thyme

Directions:

1. Firstly, the zucchini is washed.

2. Then fine noodles are cut from the zucchini with a spiral cutter.

3. Then the peppers are washed off, halved, pitted and diced.

61

4. Meanwhile, stir the thyme leaves with the pumpkin seed oil, lemon juice, oregano and a pinch of salt and pepper.

5. Now two tablespoons of olive oil are heated in a pan.

6. Now the zucchini noodles are cooked in the pan over a low heat for about three minutes.

7. After the three minutes, the oil and lemon juice mixture is added.

8. Then the trout fillets are plucked into small pieces and served on a plate with the zucchini noodles.

9. Finally, the dish is sprinkled with the pepperoni cubes and refined with a dash of lemon juice.

Sea Man's Mussels

Ingredients:

- 310 ml dry white wine
- 1 two parsley
- 1 pinch of salt, pepper and sugar
- 4 tablespoons of olive oil
- 1 baguette
- 2 kg of mussels
- 1 onion
- 6 cloves of garlic
- 520 g tomato puree

Directions:

1. Firstly, you should brush the mussels well under running water and remove any "beards" with a knife.
2. If a few clams are already open, you can tap them 2-3 times on an edge.

3. Usually they close again. If not, you should discard these clams.

4. Now the onion and garlic are finely diced and lightly sautéed in heated olive oil.

5. Then the strained tomatoes are added and simmered for a few minutes.

6. Now season the whole thing with salt, pepper and sugar, add the dry white wine and bring to the boil once.

7. Next season again and add the chopped parsley.

8. Now the prepared tomato sauce is poured boiling hot into a large saucepan.

9. Then the mussels are added to the boiling sauce.

10. Now the pot is closed with a lid and the mussels are left to cook in it for 10 minutes. Stir every now and then.

11. Once the clams open, they're done.

12. You should discard mussels that are still closed after cooking.

13. Finally, the mussels are spread over two deep plates with a little sauce.

14. A baguette, which is refined with olive oil, is ideal for this dish to dip into the sauce.

Fennel Grill Pan

Ingredients:

- 2 sprigs of rosemary

- 2 sprigs of thyme

- 4 tablespoons of olive oil

- 1 pinch of salt and pepper

- 1 bulb of fennel

- 2 tomatoes

- 2 cloves of garlic

Directions:

1. Firstly, you should make four grill bowls out of simple aluminum foil.

2. To do this, you can take a sufficiently large piece of aluminum foil, fold up the sides and put a piece of butter in it.

3. Now the fennel is cut into thin slices and distributed in the 4 aluminum foils.

4. Then the tomatoes are cut into not too thin slices and spread over the fennel.

5. Now the garlic cloves are cut into fine slices and layered on the tomato slices.

6. Now the bowls are seasoned vigorously with salt and pepper.

7. Then the herb stalks are halved and also distributed on the vegetables.

8. Next, put a spoonful of olive oil on each packet and seal the packet.

9. A pinch of herb butter is also good in the bowls next to the olive oil.

10. Now the well-sealed aluminum packs are placed on the grill for about 17 minutes.

11. Depending on how crispy you like the fennel, it's best to do a cooking test in between.

12. Finally, the finished packet is drizzled with a little olive oil.

Fluffy Tomato Soup

Ingredients:

- 4 kl canned tomatoes or 770 g fresh, finely chopped tomatoes

- 120 g black olives

- 1 sprig of basil

- 1 pinch of salt and pepper

- 120g salami

- 2 onions

- 2 tablespoons of olive oil

Directions:

1. Firstly, the salami is cut into small cubes, the onion is peeled and finely chopped and the olives are roughly chopped.

2. Next, gently fry the salami and onion in the heated oil for about three minutes.

3. After three minutes, the tomatoes are added, brought to the boil and simmered over a low heat for about 10 minutes.

4. Then the chopped olives are added and seasoned with salt, pepper and cayenne pepper.

5. Finally, the leaves are plucked from the basil, finely chopped and sprinkled over the soup for serving.

Tasty Swordfish Steaks

Ingredients:

- 1 dash of dry white wine

- 1 handful of flour

- 1 dash of lemon juice

- 2 tablespoons of olive oil

- 1 sprig of parsley

- 1 pinch of salt, pepper and cayenne

- 4 swordfish steaks

- 270 g chopped tomatoes or a can of chopped tomatoes

- 1 onion

- 4 cloves of garlic

- 4 teaspoons of capers

Directions:

1. Firstly, you should wash the swordfish steaks thoroughly, drizzle with lemon juice and let them steep for a while.

2. Next, the garlic is finely diced and the onion is cut into fine strips.

3. Now a tablespoon of olive oil is heated in a pan. Then the garlic and onions are lightly sweated in it.

4. The whole thing is then extinguished with the white wine, the tomatoes added and the sauce simmered for 10 minutes.

5. In the meantime you should pat the fish dry, season with salt, pepper and a hint of cayenne and turn it neatly in flour.

6. Now heat the remaining oil in a second pan and sear the swordfish steaks on each side for about 6-8 minutes.

7. Meanwhile the capers are added to the tomato sauce and seasoned with salt, pepper and a pinch of sugar.

8. Finally, the steaks are arranged on the tomato sauce and served sprinkled with the plucked parsley.

Arugula Salad

Ingredients:

- A medium tomato, wedged
- Black pepper and salt to taste
- 2 teaspoon rice vinegar
- 1 an avocado, halved, pitted, and sliced
- 1 tablespoon of Parmesan
- 1 cup of tomatoes cut in half
- 2 cups of baby arugula leaves
- 1 tablespoon extra virgin olive oil
- 2 tablespoons pine nuts

Directions:

1. In a wide container or bowl with a lid, add all the Ingredients:except the avocado, season with the salt and pepper, and shake well to mix.
2. Add the avocado slices before serving.

3. Transfer the arugula salad to a serving platter or plate.

Greek Salad

Ingredients:

- 1 tablespoon extra virgin olive oil

- 1 teaspoon of dried oregano

- 1 cup feta

- Olives to your liking, pitted and sliced

- Salt and black pepper to taste

- 1 large tomato, chopped

- 2 English cucumber, peeled and chopped

- 1 small onion, chopped

- 2 teaspoon lemon juice

Directions:

1. Add the tomato, onion, and cucumber to a salad bowl.
2. Sprinkle the olive oil, lemon juice, oregano, salt and pepper, and toss.

3. Crumble the feta cheese and sprinkle it and the olives over the salad.

4. Serve as desired.

Tuna Salad With A Dijon Vinaigrette

Ingredients:

For The Salad:

- 1 green onion, chopped

- 1 small red onion, chopped

- 1/2 cup olives, pitted and halved

- 1 cup of chopped parsley

- Tomato slices for serving

- 25-oz cans of tuna

- 1/2 English cucumber, chopped

- 2 small radishes, chopped

- 2 celery stalk, chopped

For The Vinaigrette:

- 1 cup virgin olive oil

- Salt, red pepper flakes (optional), and black pepper to taste

- 2 teaspoons of quality Dijon mustard

- The juice and zest of 1 lime

- 1 tablespoon of parsley, chopped

Directions:

1. In a small container, whisk the mustard, lime zest, and juice.

2. Add the olive oil, red pepper flakes, salt, and black pepper.

3. Whisk until everything combines well. Set aside.

4. For the salad, combine the tuna, chopped vegetables, olives, and parsley in a large salad bowl and mix gently.

5. Pour the Dijon Dressing: over the salad and mix again to ensure it is evenly coated.

6. Cover and refrigerate for 30 minutes.

7. Toss the salad again before serving, adding the tomato slices on the side.

8. Serve in pita pockets or over crackers.

Tabbouleh

Ingredients:

- 1 cup of finely chopped parsley

- 2 tablespoons of extra virgin olive oil

- 2 firm tomatoes, finely chopped

- 2 tablespoons of lemon/lime juice

- Lettuce leaves to serve (optional)

- Salt to taste

- 1/2 cup of extra fine bulgur wheat

- 1 English cucumber, finely chopped

- 6 mint leaves with the stems removed, washed, dried, and finely chopped

- 2 green onions, finely chopped

Directions:

1. Wash the bulgur wheat and soak it for about seven minutes. Drain well and set aside.

2. After chopping the tomatoes, place them in a colander to drain any excess juices.

3. In a salad bowl, place the chopped vegetables, add the wheat, season with salt and mix everything gently.

4. Drizzle the lime/lemon juice and olive oil over the vegetables and mix again.

5. Refrigerate for about half an hour to give the flavors time to meld.

6. Serve on a platter over some lettuce leaves and pita bread.

Packed Sardines

Ingredients:

- 2 garlic cloves, minced

- 2 tablespoons minced fresh parsley

- 2 teaspoons grated orange zest plus wedges for serving

- 3 tablespoons extra-virgin olive oil

- 8 fresh sardines (2 to 3 ounces each), scaled, gutted, head and tail on

- Salt and pepper

- 1/2 cup golden raisins, chopped fine

- 1/2 cup pine nuts, toasted and chopped fine

- 1 cup capers, rinsed and minced

- 1 cup panko bread crumbs

Directions:

1. Place oven rack to lower-middle position and pre-heat your oven to 450 degrees.

2. Coat rimmed baking sheet using aluminium foil.

3. Mix capers, raisins, pine nuts, 1 tablespoon oil, parsley, orange zest, garlic, 1/2 teaspoon salt, and 1/2 teaspoon pepper in a container.

4. Put in panko and slowly mix until blended.

5. Use a pairing knife to slit belly of fish open from gill to tail, leaving spine undamaged.

6. Gently rinse fish under cold running water and pat dry using paper towels.

7. Rub skin of sardines evenly with remaining 2 tablespoons oil and sprinkle with salt and pepper.

8. Place sardines on readied sheet, spaced 1 inch apart.

9. Stuff cavities of each sardine with 2 tablespoons filling and push on filling to help it stick; softly press fish closed.

10. Bake Until Fish Flakes Apart When Softly Poked Using Paring Knife And Filling Is Golden Brown, About Fifteen Minutes. Serve With Orange Wedges.

Provençal Anchovy Dip

Ingredients:

- 1 tablespoon minced fresh chives

- 1 teaspoon Dijon mustard

- 2 tablespoons lemon juice, plus extra for serving

- 2 tablespoons raisins

- 20 anchovy fillets (2 ounces), rinsed, patted dry, and minced

- Salt and pepper

- 1/2 cup extra-virgin olive oil, plus extra for serving

- 1/2 cup water

- 2 cup whole blanched almonds

- 1 garlic clove, minced

Directions:

1. Bring 4 cups water to boil in moderate-sized saucepan on moderate to high heat.

2. Put in almonds and cook till they become tender, approximately twenty minutes.

3. Drain and wash thoroughly.

4. Process drained almonds, anchovies, water, raisins, lemon juice, garlic, mustard, 1/2 teaspoon pepper, and 1 teaspoon salt using a food processor until a somewhat smooth paste is achieved, approximately two minutes, scraping down sides of the container as required.

5. While your food processor runs slowly put in oil and process to smooth puree, approximately two minutes.

6. Move Mixture To A Container, Mix In 2 Teaspoons Chives, And Sprinkle With Salt And Extra Lemon Juice To Taste. (Dip Will Keep Safely In A Fridge For Up To 2 Days; Bring To

Room Temperature Before You Serve.) Drizzle With The Rest Of The Chives And Extra Oil To Taste Before You Serve.

Rich Turkish Nut Dip

Ingredients:

- 1 slice hearty white sandwich bread, crusts removed, torn into 1-inch pieces

- 1 small garlic clove, minced

- 2 tablespoons lemon juice, plus extra as required

- Pinch cayenne pepper

- Salt and pepper

- 1/2 cup extra-virgin olive oil

- 2 cup water, plus extra as required

- 1 cup blanched almonds, blanched hazelnuts, pine nuts, or walnuts, toasted

Directions:

1. Using a fork, mash bread and water together in a container till it turns into a paste.

2. Process bread mixture, nuts, oil, lemon juice, garlic, 1 teaspoon salt, 1 teaspoon pepper, and cayenne using a blender until smooth, approximately two minutes.

3. Put in extra water as required until sauce is slightly thicker than consistency of heavy cream.

4. Drizzle With Salt, Pepper, And Extra Lemon Juice To Taste.

5. Serve At Room Temperature. (Sauce Will Keep Safely In A Fridge For Up To 2 Days; Bring To Room Temperature Before You Serve.)

Searing Garlic Shrimp

Ingredients:

- 1 pound medium-large shrimp (31 to 40 per pound), peeled, deveined, and tails removed

- 1 tablespoon minced fresh parsley

- 2 teaspoons sherry vinegar

- 14 garlic cloves, peeled, 2 cloves minced, 12 cloves left whole

- 1/2 teaspoon salt

- 1 cup extra-virgin olive oil

- 1 (2-inch) piece mild dried chile, approximately broken, with seeds

- 1 bay leaf

Directions:

1. Toss shrimp with minced garlic, 2 tablespoons oil, and salt in a container and allow to

marinate at room temperature for minimum half an hour or maximum 1 hour.

2. In the meantime, use the flat side of a chef's knife to smash 4 garlic cloves.

3. Heat smashed garlic and remaining 6 tablespoons oil in 12-inch frying pan over moderate to low heat, stirring intermittently, until garlic is light golden brown, four to eight minutes; allow the oil to cool to room temperature.

4. Using slotted spoon, take out and discard smashed garlic.

5. Finely cut remaining 8 garlic cloves.

6. Return frying pan with cooled oil to low heat and put in sliced garlic, bay leaf, and chile.

7. Cook, stirring intermittently, until garlic becomes soft but not browned, four to eight minutes.

8. If garlic does not begun to sizzle after 3 minutes, raise the heat to moderate to low.

9. Increase Heat To Moderate To Low And Put In Shrimp With Marinade.

10. Cook, Without Stirring, Until Oil Starts To Bubble Mildly, Approximately Two Minutes.

11. Using Tongs, Flip Shrimp And Carry On Cooking Until Almost Cooked Through, Approximately Two Minutes.

12. Increase Heat To High And Put In Vinegar And Parsley.

13. Cook, Stirring Continuously, Until Shrimp Are Cooked Through And Oil Is Bubbling Heavily, 15 To 20 Seconds.

14. Take Out And Throw Away The Bay Leaf. Serve Instantly.

Skordalia

Ingredients:

- 3 garlic cloves, minced to paste

- 3 tablespoons lemon juice

- 6 tablespoons warm water, plus extra as required

- Salt and pepper

- 1/2 cup extra-virgin olive oil

- 1/2 cup plain Greek yogurt

- 1 (10- to 12-ounce) russet potato, peeled and cut into 1-inch chunks

- 2 slices hearty white sandwich bread, crusts removed, torn into 1-inch pieces

Directions:

1. Place potato in small saucepan and put in water to cover by 1 inch.

2. Bring water to boil, then decrease heat to simmer and cook until potato becomes soft and paring knife can be inserted into potato easily, fifteen to twenty minutes.

3. Drain potato using a colander, tossing to eliminate all surplus water.

4. In the meantime, combine garlic and lemon juice in a container and allow to sit for about ten minutes. In separate medium bowl, mash bread, 1/2cup warm water, and 1 teaspoon salt till it turns into a paste with fork.

5. Move Potato To Ricer (Food Mill Fitted With Small Disk) And Process Into A Container With Bread Mixture.

6. Mix In Lemon-Garlic Mixture, Oil, Yogurt, And Remaining 2 Tablespoons Warm Water Until Thoroughly Mixed. (Sauce Will Keep Safely In A Fridge For Up To 3 Days; Bring To Room Temperature Before You Serve.) Drizzle With Salt And Pepper To Taste And Adjust

Consistency With Extra Warm Water As Required Before You Serve.

Soft And Crispy Halloumi

Ingredients:

- 2 tablespoons cornmeal

- 2 tablespoons extra-virgin olive oil

- Lemon wedges

- 1 (8-ounce) block halloumi cheese, sliced into 1-inch-thick slabs

- 1 tablespoon all-purpose flour

Directions:

1. Mix cornmeal and flour in shallow dish. Working with 1 piece of cheese at a time, coat both wide sides with cornmeal mixture, pressing to help coating stick; move to plate.

2. Heat Oil In 12-Inch Non-Stick Frying Pan Over Medium Heat Until It Starts To Shimmer.

3. Arrange Halloumi In One Layer In Frying Pan And Cook Until Golden Brown On Both Sides, 2 To 4 Minutes Each Side.

4. Move To Platter And Serve With Lemon
   Wedges.

Stuffed Dates Wrap

Ingredients:

- 12 large pitted dates, halved along the length
- 12 thin slices prosciutto, halved along the length
- 2 tablespoons extra-virgin olive oil
- Salt and pepper
- 1 cup minced fresh parsley
- 1 teaspoon grated orange zest
- 2 cup walnuts, toasted and chopped fine

Directions:

1. Mix walnuts, parsley, oil, and orange zest in a container and sprinkle with salt and pepper to taste.
2. Mound 1 large teaspoon filling into centre of each date half.
3. Wrap Prosciutto Tightly Around Dates. Serve.

Hot Asparagus Sticks

Ingredients:

- 2 tablespoons cayenne pepper sauce
- A pinch of salt and black pepper
- 1 cup water
- 1 and 2 pounds asparagus, trimmed
- 2 tablespoons olive oil

Directions:

1. In A Bowl, Mix The Asparagus With The Other Ingredients:Except The Water And Toss.
2. Put The Water In Your Instant Pot, Add The Steamer Basket, Put The Asparagus Sticks Inside, Put The Lid On And Cook On High For 6 Minutes.
3. Release The Pressure Fast For 5 Minutes, Arrange The Asparagus On A Platter And Serve.

Asparagus Couscous Salad

Ingredients:

- 1 bunch asparagus

- 2 cups arugula

- 1 lemon, juiced

- Salt and pepper to taste

- 1 cup couscous

- 1 cup vegetable stock, hot

- 1 teaspoon dried tarragon

Directions:

1. Combine the couscous and stock in a bowl. Cover with a lid and allow to soak up all the liquid.
2. Fluff up the couscous with a fork then allow it to cool down.

3. Using a vegetable peeler, peel the asparagus into fine ribbons and place them in your salad bowl.

4. Add the rest of the Ingredients:and season with salt and pepper.

5. Serve the salad as fresh as possible.

Mango Salsa

Ingredients:

- 1 cup cherry tomatoes, cubed

- 1 cup avocado, peeled, pitted and cubed

- A pinch of salt and black pepper

- 1 tablespoon olive oil

- 1/2 cup tomato puree

- 1 cup kalamata olives, pitted and sliced

- 2 mangoes, peeled and cubed

- 1 tablespoon sweet paprika

- 2 garlic cloves, minced

- 2 tablespoons cilantro, chopped

- 1 tablespoon spring onions, chopped

Directions:

1. In Your Instant Pot, Combine The Mangoes
   With The Paprika And The Rest Of The

Ingredients:Except The Cilantro, Put The Lid On And Cook On High For 5 Minutes.

2. Release The Pressure Fast For 5 Minutes, Divide The Mix Into Small Bowls, Sprinkle The Cilantro On Top And Serve.

Pork Bites

Ingredients:

- 2 tablespoons water

- 1 tablespoon sweet paprika

- 2 tablespoons tomato sauce

- 1 tablespoon rosemary, chopped

- 1 pound pork roast, cubed and browned

- 1 tablespoon Italian seasoning

- 1 cup beef stock

Directions:

1. In Your Instant Pot, Combine The Pork Cubes With The Seasoning And The Rest Of The Ingredients:Except The Rosemary, Toss, Put The Lid On And Cook On High For 30 Minutes.

2. Release The Pressure Naturally For 10 Minutes, Arrange The Pork Cubes On A

Platter, Sprinkle The Rosemary On Top And Serve.

Tomato Greek Salad

Ingredients:

- 1 red onion, sliced

- 1/2 cup parsley, chopped

- Salt and pepper to taste

- 1 tablespoon balsamic vinegar

- 2 tablespoons extra virgin olive oil

- 1 pound tomatoes, cubed

- 1 cucumber, sliced

- 1 cup black olives

- 1/2 cup sun-dried tomatoes, chopped

Directions:

1. Combine the tomatoes, cucumber, black olives, sun-dried tomatoes, onion and parsley in a bowl.

2. Add salt and pepper to taste then stir in the vinegar and olive oil.

3. Mix well and serve the salad fresh.

Fresh Mediterranean Salad

Ingredients:

- 1 cup chopped parsley

- 1/2 cup chopped cilantro

- 1/2 cup sliced almonds

- 1 lemon, juiced

- 1 teaspoon dried oregano

- 1 tablespoon balsamic vinegar

- 2 tablespoons extra virgin olive oil

- Salt and pepper to taste

- 1 pound tomatoes, sliced

- 1 cucumber, sliced

- 1 fennel bulb, sliced

- 1 red onion, sliced

Directions:

1. Combine the tomatoes and the remaining Ingredients:in a salad bowl.
2. Season with salt and pepper as needed and mix gently.
3. Serve the salad as fresh as possible.

Crunchy Mediterranean Salad

Ingredients:

- 1 red onion, sliced

- 2 tablespoons red wine vinegar

- Salt and pepper to taste

- 2 tablespoons pine nuts

- 1 tablespoons sliced almonds

- 1 can cannellini beans, drained

- 1 cup cherry tomatoes, halved

- 1 cucumber, diced

- 1 cup chopped parsley

- 1 red bell pepper, cored and diced

- 1 garlic clove, chopped

Directions:

1. Combine the cannellini beans, tomatoes, cucumber, parsley, bell pepper, garlic, onion and vinegar in a bowl.
2. Add salt and pepper to taste and mix well.
3. Top the salad with pine nuts and sliced almonds.
4. Serve the salad fresh.

Grilled Chicken Salad

Ingredients:

- 1 cup cherry tomatoes, halved

- 1/2 cup green olives

- 1 cucumber, sliced

- 1 lemon, juiced

- 2 tablespoons extra virgin olive oil

- Salt and pepper to taste

- 2 chicken fillets

- 1 teaspoon dried oregano

- 1 teaspoon dried basil

- 2 tablespoons olive oil

- 2 cups arugula leaves

Directions:

1. Season the chicken with salt, pepper, oregano and basil then drizzle it with olive oil.

2. Heat a grill pan over medium flame then place the chicken on the grill.

3. Cook on each side until browned then cut into thin strips.

4. Combine the chicken with the rest of the Ingredients:and mix gently.

5. Adjust the taste with salt and pepper and serve the salad as fresh as possible.

Smoky Eggplant Balsamic Salad

Ingredients:

- 1 teaspoon smoked paprika

- 2 tablespoons sherry vinegar

- 2 cups mixed greens

- 2 eggplants, sliced

- 2 tablespoons extra virgin olive oil

- 2 garlic cloves, minced

- Salt and pepper to taste

Directions:

1. Season the eggplant slices with salt and pepper.
2. Mix the oil with garlic and paprika then brush this mixture over the eggplant slices.
3. Heat a grill pan over medium flame then place the eggplant on the grill.

113

4. Cook on each side until browned then transfer the vegetable in a salad bowl.
5. Add the sherry vinegar and greens and serve the salad fresh.

Polenta Roasted Vegetable Salad

Ingredients:

- 1 teaspoon dried oregano

- 1 teaspoon dried basil

- 2 tablespoons balsamic vinegar

- 2 tablespoons extra virgin olive oil

- Salt and pepper to taste

- 1 1/4 cups water

- 1 cup polenta flour

- 1 zucchini, sliced

- 2 eggplants, sliced

- 2 tomatoes, sliced

Directions:

1. Combine the water with a pinch of salt and bring it to a boil.

2. Stir in the polenta flour and mix while cooking for a few minutes.
3. Pour the polenta in a square pan and level it well then allow to cool down and cut into small cubes.
4. Cook the vegetables on a heated grill pan until browned then place them in a large salad bowl with the polenta cubes.
5. Add the vinegar, oil, oregano, basil, salt and pepper.
6. Mix gently and serve the salad fresh.

Artichoke Tuna Salad

Ingredients:

- ¼ cup green olives, sliced

- 1 lemon, juiced

- 1 tablespoon Dijon mustard

- 2 tablespoons extra virgin olive oil

- 1 jar artichoke hearts, drained and chopped

- 1 can water tuna, drained

- 2 arugula leaves

- 2 tablespoons pine nuts

- Salt and pepper to taste

Directions:

1. Combine the artichoke hearts, tuna, green olives, arugula and pine nuts in a salad bowl.
2. For the Dressing:, mix the lemon juice, mustard and oil.

3. Drizzle the Dressing: over the salad and serve the salad as fresh as possible.

Smoked Salmon Lentil Salad

Ingredients:

- 1 red pepper, chopped

- 1 red onion, chopped

- Salt and pepper to taste

- 4 oz. smoked salmon, shredded

- 1 lemon, juiced

- 1 cup green lentils, rinsed

- 2 cups vegetable stock

- 1 cup chopped parsley

- 2 tablespoons chopped cilantro

Directions:

1. Combine the lentils and stock in a saucepan.

2. Cook on low heat for 15-20 minutes or until all the liquid has been absorbed completely.

3. Transfer the lentils in a salad bowl and add the parsley, cilantro, red pepper and onion. Season with salt and pepper.
4. Add the smoked salmon and lemon juice and mix well.
5. Serve the salad fresh.

Chicken Wings Platter

Ingredients:

- 1 teaspoon smoked paprika

- 1 tablespoon cilantro, chopped

- 1 tablespoon chives, chopped

- 2 pounds chicken wings

- 1 cup tomato sauce

- A pinch of salt and black pepper

Directions:

1. In Your Instant Pot, Combine The Chicken Wings With The Sauce And The Rest Of The Ingredients, Stir, Put The Lid On And Cook On High For 20 Minutes.

2. Release The Pressure Naturally For 10 Minutes, Arrange The Chicken Wings On A Platter And Serve As An Appetizer.

Beef Stroganoff

Ingredients:

- 2 tablespoons tomato paste

- 1 cup sliced mushroom

- 2 garlic cloves, minced

- 1 onion, chopped

- 1 tablespoon almond flour

- 3 tablespoon olive oil

- 2 cups of beef strip

- 1/2 teaspoon pepper

- 1/2 teaspoon salt

- 2 cups zucchini noodles

- 2 cups beef broth

- 3 tablespoons Worcestershire sauce

Directions:

1. In a bowl mix the beef strips, flour, salt, and pepper.

2. Coat the beef strips with flour and seasoning.

3. Set your instant pot on low heat and low pressure, with a cook time of 10-minutes.

4. Cook your meat for 10-minutes.

5. Place the remaining Ingredients:into the pot and set for an additional 18-minutes.

6. When the cook time is completed, release the pressure naturally for 10-minutes.

7. Serve with some zoodles.

Lamb & Feta Meatballs

Ingredients:

- 6-ounce can of tomato sauce

- 1/2 teaspoon black pepper

- 1 teaspoon salt

- 1 teaspoon oregano, dried

- 1 tablespoon water

- 1 tablespoon mint, fresh, chopped

- 2 lbs. ground lamb

- 4 garlic cloves, minced

- 1 (28-ounce) can of crushed tomatoes

- 2 tablespoons olive oil

- 2 tablespoons chopped parsley

- 1 cup breadcrumbs

- 1 cup crumbled feta cheese

- 1 onion, chopped

- 1 green bell pepper, chopped

- 1 beaten egg

Directions:

1. In a bowl, mix breadcrumbs, egg, lamb, mint, parsley, feta, water, half of the minced garlic, pepper and salt.

2. Mold into 1-inch balls using your hands.

3. Set your instant pot to the sauté mode, add oil and heat.

4. Add the onion and bell pepper to hot oil and cook for 2-minutes before the rest of the garlic.

5. After about 1-minute add the crushed tomatoes with their liquid, the tomato sauce, and oregano.

6. Sprinkle with salt and pepper.

7. Close and secure the pot lid, select Manual mode, on high, with a cook time of 8-minutes.

8. When the cook time is completed, release the pressure using quick-release.

9. Serve the meatballs with parsley and more cheese!

Beef Bourguignon

Ingredients:

- 2 tablespoons fresh thyme

- 2 teaspoons rock salt

- 2 garlic cloves, minced

- 1 large peeled and sliced red onion

- 5 medium-sized carrots

- 1 lb of stewing steak

- 1 lb. of bacon

- 1 tablespoon olive oil

- 1 cup beef broth

- 2 teaspoon ground black pepper

- 2 tablespoons fresh parsley, chopped

Directions:

1. Set your instant pot to the sautė mode, add 1 tablespoon of olive oil.

2. Allow oil to heat, and then add the beef and brown it.

3. Slice the cooked bacon into strips alongside the onion in your pot.

4. Add remaining Ingredients:and stir.

5. Close and secure the lid, set on Manual, on high, for a cook time of 30-minutes.

6. When the cook time is completed, release the pressure naturally for 10-minutes.

7. Serve warm and enjoy!

Instant Pot Beef Stew

Ingredients:

- 1 tablespoon tomato paste

- 1 teaspoon onion powder

- 1 teaspoon paprika

- 1 teaspoon pepper

- 2 tablespoons arrowroot flour

- Worcestershire sauce

- 16-ounces of tenderloin cut

- 1 piece of chopped onion

- 3 Yukon gold potatoes, chopped up

- 1 zucchini, chopped

- 1 cup carrots, chopped

- 2 cups beef broth

- 2 teaspoon sea salt

- 1 piece of bay leaf

Directions:

1. Set your instant pot to the sautè mode, add the oil and heat it.

2. Add the tenderloin in the oil.

3. Saute them until the meat is well cooked and no longer pink.

4. Add the vegetables and stir in the broth, with seasoning.

5. Close and secure the lid, set to Stew/Meat mode, with a cook time of 35-minutes.

6. Once cook time is completed, release the pressure naturally for 10-minutes.

7. Ladle 1/2 of the liquid into a bowl and mix arrowroot flour with it, making a slurry.

8. Add the slurry back into the instant pot and stir.

9. Season a bit with salt, serve hot and enjoy!

Simple Beef Short Ribs

Ingredients:

- 1 cup water

- 1 quartered onion

- Generous amount of kosher salt

- 4lbs. beef short ribs

- 1 tablespoon of beef fat

- 3 cloves garlic

Directions:

1. Season the beef ribs with salt all over.

2. In a skillet over medium heat add oil and allow it to heat up.

3. Add the ribs to skillet and brown them.

4. Add the onion, garlic, and water.

5. Transfer the mixture to your instant pot and stir.

6. Close and secure the lid, set on Manual mode, on high, with a cook time of 35-minutes.
7. Release the pressure naturally for 10-minutes.
8. Serve warm.

Chicken & Tomato Soup

Ingredients:

- 15-ounces tomatoes, diced

- 1 teaspoon oregano, dried

- 1 teaspoon thyme, dried

- 1 tablespoon garlic, minced

- 1 medium onion, chopped

- 1 lb. lean ground chicken

- 1 tablespoon olive oil

- Black pepper to taste

- Salt to taste

- 15-ounces chicken broth

Directions:

1. Set your instant pot to the sauté mode, add the oil and heat it.

2. Cook chicken until the meat turns brown.

3. Add onion, thyme, garlic, and oregano and cook for 3-minutes.
4. Add the tomatoes and chicken broth and close the pot lid.
5. Set the pot on the SOUP mode and cook for 30-minutes.
6. When the cooking is completed, release the pressure using the quick-release. Serve soup warm.

Chicken Chili From Instant Pot

Ingredients:

- 1 tablespoon oregano

- 2 tablespoons chili powder

- 14-ounces tomatoes, diced

- 2 jalapenos, minced

- 1 teaspoon black pepper

- ¼ teaspoon cayenne

- 2 lbs. ground chicken

- 2 tablespoons olive oil

- 2 red onions, diced

- 10 garlic cloves, minced

- 8 carrots, chopped

- 5 celery stalks, chopped

- 2 bell peppers, chopped

- 2 teaspoons salt

- 1 tablespoon cumin

Directions:

1. Set your instant pot to the sautė mode, add the oil and heat it.

2. Add the oil and garlic and sautė them for a few minutes.

3. Add the chicken and brown the chicken.

4. Place the remaining Ingredients:into the pot and place the lid on the pot.

5. Set on the Bean/Chili mode, and it will automatically cook for 30-minutes.

6. When cook time is over, release the pressure naturally for 10-minutes.

7. Garnish with fresh chopped cilantro and serve warm.

Chicken Soup

Ingredients:

- 1 small yellow onion, diced

- 1 medium rutabaga, diced

- 1 large parsnip, diced

- 2 medium carrots, diced

- 2 large celery ribs, sliced

- 1.5 lbs. chicken drumsticks

- 1-quart chicken stock

- 1 teaspoon cracked black pepper

- 2 bay leaves

Directions:

1. Add all the Ingredients:into an instant pot and pour the chicken stock over them.

2. Close the lid to the pot, set pot on the SOUP setting.

3. Once the cook time is completed, release the pressure naturally.

4. Remove the chicken pieces and bones.

5. Transfer meat back to the pot and adjust seasoning if needed. Serve the soup warm.

Italian Roasted Vegetables

Ingredients:

- 11 chopped garlic cloves

- 1 tsp dried thyme

- Salt to taste

- Shredded Parmesan cheese

- Black pepper to taste

- 1 tbsp dried oregano

- Red pepper flakes to taste

- 8 oz mushrooms

- 12 oz Campari tomatoes

- Extra virgin olive as required

- 3 sliced zucchinis

- 12 oz sliced baby potatoes

Directions:

1. Add salt, mushrooms, olive oil, pepper, veggies, oregano, garlic, and thyme in a mixing bowl and toss well. Set aside.

2. Roast potatoes in a preheated oven at 425 degrees for 10 minutes.

3. Mix the mushroom mixture with baked potatoes and bake for another 20 minutes.

4. Garnish with cheese and pepper flakes and serve.

White Bean Salad

Ingredients:

- 1 tbsp of lemon juice

- Salt to taste

- Zested of one lemon

- Black pepper to taste

- 1 tsp Sumac

- Feta cheese

- 1 tsp Za'atar

- 1 tsp Aleppo

- Olive oil

- 2o oz white beans

- 10 oz halved cherry tomatoes

- 2 chopped English cucumber

- 5 chopped onion

- 18 chopped mint leaves

- 1 cup chopped parsley

Directions:

1. Combine all the Ingredients:in a large salad bowl and toss well to mix everything evenly.
2. Serve and enjoy it.

Roasted Cauliflower With Lemon And Cumin

Ingredients:

- 1 tbsp ground sumac

- 1 tbsp ground cumin

- 1 tsp garlic powder

- Black pepper to taste

- 11 oz cauliflower

- 1 tbsp of lemon juice

- 1/3 cup olive oil

- Salt to taste

- Zest of one lemon

Directions:

1. Mix all the Ingredients:in a large mixing bowl.

2. Transfer the cauliflower to a baking tray and bake in a preheated oven at 425 degrees for 25 minutes. Serve and enjoy it.

Tabbouleh Salad

Ingredients:

- 5 chopped green onions

- 13 chopped mint leaves

- Salt to taste

- 4 tbsp extra virgin olive oil

- 4 tbsp lime juice

- Romaine lettuce leaves to garnishing

- 1 cup bulgur wheat

- 2 chopped English cucumber

- 4 chopped tomatoes

- 3 chopped parsley

Directions:

1. Soak bulgur for 10 minutes in water.

2. Drain to remove all the excess water and keep it aside.

3. Now, mix all the Ingredients:in a large salad bowl and place them for 30 minutes in the refrigerator to get the best results.

Watermelon Salad

Ingredients:

- 1 chopped watermelon

- Watermelon Salad

- 2 tbsp lime juice

- 2 chopped English cucumber

- 15 chopped basil leaves

- 15 chopped mint leaves

- 1 cup feta cheese

- Honey Vinaigrette

- 2 tbsp extra virgin olive oil

- 2 tbsp honey

- 2 pinch of salt

Directions:

1. In a bowl, combine watermelon, herbs, and cucumber and set aside.

2. In another bowl, mix oil, salt, honey, and lemon juice and pour the Dressing: into a watermelon bowl.
3. Toss well and serve.

Loaded Chickpea Salad

Ingredients:

- Salt to taste

- 1 chopped English cucumber

- 1 cup chopped parsley

- 2 chopped small red onion

- 1 cup chopped dill

- Olive oil

- 3 sliced eggplant

- 1 cup cooked chickpeas

- 4 diced Roma tomatoes

- 3 tbsp Za'atar spice

Garlic Vinaigrette:

- 1/3 cup extra virgin olive oil

- 2 tbsp lime juice

- Two chopped garlic cloves

148

- Salt to taste

- Black pepper to taste

Directions:

1. Season eggplant with salt and set aside for 30 minutes.

2. Dry eggplant and cook in olive oil for five minutes from each side.

3. When the eggplant has turned brown from both sides, remove the pan from the flame and keep it aside.

4. In a bowl, combine cucumber, onions, tomatoes, dill, zaatar, chickpeas, parsley, and mix well.

5. Place all the Dressing: Ingredients:in a bowl and toss well.

6. Transfer cooked eggplant and chickpeas mixture in one large bowl and poured the Dressing: over them.

7. Serve and enjoy it.

Baked Zucchini With Thyme And Parmesan

Ingredients:

- 1/4 tsp garlic powder
- Kosher salt to taste
- 1/2 tsp dried basil
- Black pepper to taste
- 2 tbsp chopped parsley
- Four sliced zucchinis
- 1/2 tsp dried thyme
- 1/2 cup shredded Parmesan cheese
- 1/2 tsp dried oregano
- 2 tbsp olive oil

Directions:

1. Mix all the Ingredients:in a large bowl except zucchini.

2. Make a layer of zucchini over a baking sheet sprayed with oil.
3. Transfer the cheese mixture over zucchini and pour olive oil over them.
4. Bake in a preheated oven at 350 degrees for 15 minutes, followed by broiling for three minutes.
5. Serve and enjoy it.

Baba Ganoush

Ingredients:

- 1 tsp cayenne pepper

- Pepper to taste

- 1 tsp sumac for garnishing

- Parsley leaves for garnishing

- Toasted pine nuts for garnishing

- 2 eggplant

- 1 tbsp Greek yogurt

- olive oil

- 2 tbsp tahini paste

- 1 tbsp lime juice

- 2 garlic clove

- Salt to taste

Directions:

1. Make slits in eggplant's skin.

2. Place eggplant skin side upwards in a baking tray.

3. Spray olive oil over eggplant.

4. Bake in a preheated oven at 425 degrees for 40 minutes.

5. Scoop the inner flesh of eggplant out and shift in a food processor.

6. Add garlic, cayenne, yogurt, lime juice, salt, tahini, sumac, pepper, and blend.

7. The baba ganoush is ready.

8. You can refrigerator for better results for 60 minutes and sprinkle oil, sumac, parsley, and nuts and serve.

Salmon Fish Sticks

Ingredients:

Fish Sticks:

- 1/4 tsp salt

- 1/4 tsp black pepper

- 2 lb salmon fillet

First Coating:

- 1 cup almond meal

- 1/2 tsp sea salt

- 1/4 tsp black pepper

- 1/2 tsp garlic powder

- 1/2 tsp dried thyme

Second Coating:

- Third coating

- 3 eggs

- 1/2 tsp salt

- 2/3 cup chickpea flour

Dipping Sauce:

- 1 tbsp Dijon mustard

- 1/2 tsp dill

- 1/8 tsp garlic powder

- 1/4 tsp salt

- 1/4 cup Greek yogurt

- 1 tsp lemon juice

Directions:

1. Whisk all the Ingredients:for the dipping sauce list in a bowl and set aside.

2. The dipping sauce is ready.

3. Mix garlic, thyme, and almond meal in a bowl. The first coating is ready.

4. Add chickpea flour in another bowl. The second coating is ready.

5. Beat the eggs in another bowl. Set aside.

6. Sprinkle pepper and salt over sliced fish with removed skin.

7. First, coat the fish with chickpea flour, followed by coating with egg and almond meal coating.

8. Aline coated fish pieces in a baking sheet covered with parchment paper.

9. Bake in a preheated oven at 400 degrees for 18 minutes.

10. Serve baked fish with dipping sauce and serve.

Baked Falafel

Ingredients:

- 15 oz chickpeas

- 4 cloves garlic

- 1/4 cup chopped onion

- 1 tsp ground cumin

- 3/4 tsp salt

- 1 tsp coriander

- 2 pinch of cayenne

- 3 tbsp oat flour

- 1/2 cup parsley

- 2 tsp lemon juice

- 1/2 tsp baking soda

- 1 tbsp olive oil

Directions:

1. Blend all the Ingredients: except oat flour and baking soda in a food processor to get roughly a blended mixture.
2. Transfer the mixture to a bowl and add oat flour and baking soda.
3. Using hands, mix the dough well.
4. Make patties out of the falafel mixture and set aside for 15 minutes.
5. Bake the falafel patties in a preheated oven at 375 degrees for 12 minutes and serve.

Green Smoothie

Ingredients:

- 2 Cup Organic Almond Milk

- 1 Tablespoon Almonds, Chopped

- 1 Cup Of Water

- 2 Cups Spinach

- 2 Cups Kale

- 1 Cup Bok Choy

Directions:

1. Place All Ingredients: In The Blender And Blend Until You Get A Smooth Mixture.

2. Pour The Smoothie In The Serving Glasses. Add Ice Cubes If Desired.

Simple And Quick Steak

Ingredients:

- 1 Lb Steak, Quality - Cut Salt And Freshly
- Cracked Black Pepper

Directions:

1. Switch On The Air Fryer, Set Frying Basket In It, Then Set Its Temperature To 385°F And Let Preheat.

2. Meanwhile, Prepare The Steaks, And For This, Season Steaks With Salt And Freshly Cracked Black Pepper On Both Sides.

3. When Air Fryer Has Preheated, Add Prepared Steaks In The Fryer Basket, Shut It With Lid And Cook For 15 Minutes. When Done, Transfer Steaks To A Dish And Then Serve Immediately.

4. For Meal Prepping, Evenly Divide The Steaks Between Two Heatproof Containers, Close

Them With Lid And Refrigerate For Up To 3
Days Until Ready To Serve.

5. When Ready To Eat, Reheat Steaks Into The
    Microwave Until Hot And Then Serve.

Almonds Crusted Rack Of Lamb With Rosemary

Ingredients:

- 1 Small Organic Egg

- 1 Tbsp Breadcrumbs

- 2 Oz Almonds, Finely Chopped

- 1 Tbsp Fresh Rosemary, Chopped

- 1 Garlic Clove, Minced

- 1 Tbsp Olive Oil

- Salt And Freshly Cracked Black Pepper

- 2 Lb Rack Of Lamb

Directions:

1. Switch On The Oven And Set Its Temperature To 350°F, And Let It Preheat. Meanwhile, Take A Baking Tray, Grease It With Oil, And Set Aside Until Required.

2. Mix Garlic, Oil, Salt, And Freshly Cracked Black Pepper In A Bowl And Coat The Rack Of Lamb With This Garlic, Rub On All Sides.

3. Crack The Egg In A Bowl, Whisk Until Blended, And Set Aside Until Required.

4. Place Breadcrumbs In Another Dish, Add Almonds And Rosemary And Stir Until Mixed.

5. Dip The Seasoned Rack Of Lamb With Egg, Dredge With The Almond Mixture Until Evenly Coated On All Sides And Then Place It Onto The Prepared Baking Tray.

6. When The Oven Has Preheated, Place The Rack Of Lamb In It, And Cook For 35 Minutes Until Thoroughly Cooked.

7. When Done, Take Out The Baking Tray, Transfer Rack Of Lamb Onto A Dish, And Serve Straight Away.

8. For Meal Prep, Cut Rack Of Lamb Into Pieces, Evenly Divide The Lamb Between Two Heatproof Containers, Close Them With Lid

And Refrigerate For Up To 3 Days Until Ready To Serve. When Ready To Eat, Reheat Rack Of Lamb In The Microwave Until Hot And Then Serve.

Cheesy Eggs In Avocado

Ingredients:

- 1/2 Cup Shredded Cheddar Cheese Salt And Freshly Cracked Black Pepper

- 1 Tbsp Olive Oil

- 1 Medium Avocado 2 Organic Eggs

Directions:

1. Switch On The Oven, Then Set Its Temperature To 425°F, And Let Preheat.

2. Meanwhile, Prepare The Avocados And For This, Cut The Avocado In Half And Remove Its Pit. Take Two Muffin Tins, Grease Them With Oil, And Then Add An Avocado Half Into Each Tin.

3. Crack An Egg Into Each Avocado Half, Season Well With Salt And Freshly Cracked Black Pepper, And Then Sprinkle Cheese On Top.

4. When The Oven Has Preheated, Place The Muffin Tins In The Oven And Bake For 15 Minutes Until Cooked. When Done, Take Out The Muffin Tins, Transfer The Avocados Baked Organic Eggs To A Dish, And Then Serve Them.

Bacon, Vegetable And Parmesan Combo

Ingredients:

- 1 Of Medium Green Bell Pepper, Deseeded, Chopped

- 1 Scallion, Chopped

- 1/2 Cup Grated Parmesan Cheese

- 1 Tbsp Olive Oil

- 2 Slices Of Bacon, Thick-Cut

- 1 Tbsp Mayonnaise

Directions:

1. Switch On The Oven, Then Set Its Temperature To 375°F And Let It Preheat.

2. Meanwhile, Take A Baking Dish, Grease It With Oil, And Add Slices Of Bacon In It.

3. Spread Mayonnaise On Top Of The Bacon, Then Top With Bell Peppers And Scallions,

Sprinkle With Parmesan Cheese And Bake For About 25 Minutes Until Cooked Thoroughly.

4. When Done, Take Out The Baking Dish And Serve Immediately.

5. For Meal Prepping, Wrap Bacon In A Plastic Sheet And Refrigerate For Up To 2 Days.

6. When Ready To Eat, Reheat Bacon In The Microwave And Then Serve.

Four-Cheese Zucchini Noodles With Basil Pesto

Ingredients:

- 1 Tsp Cracked Black Pepper

- 2 1/8 Tsp Ground Nutmeg

- 1/8 Cup Basil Pesto

- 1 Cup Shredded Mozzarella Cheese

- 1 Tbsp Olive Oil

- 4 Cups Zucchini Noodles

- 4 Oz Mascarpone Cheese

- 1/8 Cup Romano Cheese

- 2 Tbsp Grated Parmesan Cheese

- 1/2 Tsp Salt

Directions:

1. Switch On The Oven, Then Set Its Temperature To 400°F And Let It Preheat.

2. Meanwhile, Place Zucchini Noodles In A Heatproof Bowl And Microwave At High Heat Setting For 3 Minutes, Set Aside Until Required.

3. Take Another Heatproof Bowl, Add All Cheeses In It, Except For Mozzarella, Season With Salt, Black Pepper And Nutmeg, And Microwave At High Heat Setting For 1 Minute Until Cheese Has Melted.

4. Whisk The Cheese Mixture, Add Cooked Zucchini Noodles In It Along With Basil Pesto And Mozzarella Cheese And Fold Until Well Mixed.

5. Take A Casserole Dish, Grease It With Oil, Add Zucchini Noodles Mixture In It, And Then Bake For 10 Minutes Until Done. Serve Straight Away.

Baked Eggs With Cheddar And Beef

Ingredients:

- 2 Organic Eggs

- 2oz Shredded Cheddar Cheese

- 1 Tbsp Olive Oil

- 3 Oz Ground Beef, Cooked

Directions:

1. Switch On The Oven, Then Set Its Temperature To 390°F And Let It Preheat.

2. Meanwhile, Take A Baking Dish, Grease It With Oil, Add Spread Cooked Beef In The Bottom, Then Make Two Holes In It And Crack An Organic Egg Into Each Hole.

3. Sprinkle Cheese On Top Of Beef And Eggs And Bake For 20 Minutes Until Beef Has Cooked And Eggs Have Set.

4. When Done, Let Baked Eggs Cool For 5 Minutes And Then Serve Straight Away.

5. For Meal Prepping, Wrap Baked Eggs In Foil And Refrigerate For Up To Two Days. When Ready To Eat, Reheat Baked Eggs In The Microwave And Then Serve.

Heavenly Egg Bake With Blackberry

Ingredients:

- 1 Tbsp Unsalted Butter

- 5 Organic Eggs

- 1 Tbsp Olive Oil

- 1 Cup Fresh Blackberries

- Black Pepper To Taste

- Chopped Rosemary 1 Tsp Lime Zest

- 1 Tsp Salt

- 1/2 Tsp Vanilla Extract, Unsweetened

- 1 Tsp Grated Ginger

- 3 Tbsp Coconut Flour

Directions:

1. Switch On The Oven, Then Set Its Temperature To 350°F And Let It Preheat.

2. Meanwhile, Place All The Ingredients:In A Blender, Reserving The Berries And Pulse For 2 To 3 Minutes Until Well Blended And Smooth.

3. Take Four Silicon Muffin Cups, Grease Them With Oil, Evenly Distribute The Blended Batter In The Cups, Top With Black Pepper And Bake For 15 Minutes Until Cooked Through And The Top Has Golden Brown.

4. When Done, Let Blueberry Egg Bake Cool In The Muffin Cups For 5 Minutes, Then Take Them Out, Cool Them On A Wire Rack And Then Serve.

5. For Meal Prepping, Wrap Each Egg Bake With Aluminum Foil And Freeze For Up To 3 Days.

6. When Ready To Eat, Reheat Blueberry Egg Bake In The Microwave And Then Serve.

Protein-Packed Blender Pancakes

Ingredients:

- 1/2 Tsp Cinnamon

- 2oz Cream Cheese, Soften

- 1 Tsp Unsalted Butter

- 2 Organic Eggs

- 1 Scoop Protein Powder Salt To Taste

Directions:

1. Crack The Eggs In A Blender, Add Remaining Ingredients:Except For Butter And Pulse For 2 Minutes Until Well Combined And Blended.

2. Take A Skillet Pan, Place It Over Medium Heat, Add Butter And When It Melts, Pour In Prepared Batter, Spread It Evenly, And Cook For 4 To 5 Minutes Per Side Until Cooked Through And Golden Brown. Serve Straight Away.

Blueberry And Vanilla Scones

Ingredients:

- 1 Cup Stevia

- 2 Tsp Vanilla Extract, Unsweetened

- 2 Cup Fresh Raspberries

- 1 Tbsp Olive Oil

- 2 Cup Almond Flour

- 3 Organic Eggs, Beaten

- 2 Tsp Baking Powder

Directions:

1. Switch On The Oven, Then Set Its Temperature To 375 °F And Let It Preheat.

2. Take A Large Bowl, Add Flour And Eggs In It, Stir In Baking Powder, Stevia, And Vanilla Until Combined And Then Fold In Berries Until Mixed.

3. Take A Baking Dish, Grease It With Oil, Scoop The Prepared Batter On It With An Ice Cream Scoop And Bake For 10 Minutes Until Done.

4. When Done, Transfer Scones On A Wire Rack, Cool Them Completely, And Then Serve.

Mediterranean Oven Vegetables

Ingredients:

- 170 g cherry tomatoes

- 1 onion

- 6 cloves of garlic

- 5 tablespoons of olive oil

- 1 pinch of salt, pepper, caraway seeds, paprika powder, thyme, marjoram, oregano and rosemary

- 520 g potatoes

- 430 g pointed peppers

- 120 g sheep cheese

- 220 g mushrooms

Directions:

1. Firstly, a pan with a good amount of olive oil is placed on top and the washed, peeled and halved potatoes are briefly tossed through.

178

2. Meanwhile, The Pointed Peppers Are Pitted, Halved And Briefly Added.

3. The Mixture Is Then Refined With The Herbs And Placed In An Ovenproof Dish.

4. Now Quarter The Tomatoes, Halve The Mushrooms And Cut The Feta Into Cubes.

5. The Onion Is Also Cut Into Rings And The Garlic Is Peeled.

6. Now All The Ingredients:For The Potatoes And Pointed Peppers Can Be Put Into The Mold, Stirred And Seasoned With Sea Salt, Pepper, Caraway Seeds And Hot Paprika Powder.

7. The Dish Can Now Be Put In The Oven For About 30 Minutes At 200 ° C.

8. When the potatoes are done, the finished oven vegetables can be served.

Vegetable Plaice With Mediterranean Gratin

Ingredients:

- 60 g parmesan cheese

- 4 tbsp chives, thyme and parsley

- 1 onion

- 1 dash of lemon juice

- 1 clove of garlic

- 1 pinch of salt and pepper

- 10 plaice fillets

- 2 eggplants

- 2 peppers

- 125 ml vegetable stock

- 2 tbsp pesto

Directions:

1. Firstly, the fresh plaice fillet is rinsed under cold water, patted dry and then marinated with salt, pepper and lemon juice.

2. Now Cut The Eggplants, Peppers And Zucchini Into Small Cubes, The Onions Into Thin Rings And The Garlic Finely Chopped.

3. Next, Put The Olive Oil In A Pan.

4. The Onion And Garlic Are Steamed In It, The Remaining Vegetables Are Added And Steamed For 2-3 Minutes.

5. After The Steaming, The Whole Thing Is Then Extinguished With The Vegetable Stock And Simmered For About 7 Minutes.

6. After The Broth And Its Contents Have Simmered For 5 Minutes, Add The Finely Chopped Herbs And Stir In.

7. Finally, The Broth Is Refined With Salt And Pepper.

8. Then The Vegetables Are Placed In A Greased Baking Dish.

9. Now The Plaice Fillet Is Coated With Pesto (Freshly Made Or Bought), Rolled Up And Placed With The Open Side Down On The Vegetables.

10. Finally, the plaice rolls are coated again with pesto, sprinkled with a lot of parmesan and baked at 200 ° for 33 minutes.

Thin Lamb Chops With Beetroot

Ingredients:

- 1 clove of garlic

- 1 tbsp rapeseed oil

- 1 tbsp olive oil

- 1 pinch of salt and pepper

- 6 lamb chops

- 320 g beetroot

- 1 onion

- 220 g of grainy cream cheese

Directions:

1. Firstly, the lamb chops are washed off, dried and then seasoned with a pinch of salt and pepper.

2. Now The Chops Are Seared On High Heat On A Grill Pan / Pan On Each Side For 3 Minutes.

3. You Can Then Keep The Lamb Chops Warm In The Oven At 80 Degrees Celsius.

4. Meanwhile, The Beetroot Is Cut Into Thin Slices And The Onion Is Peeled And Diced.

5. Now A Tablespoon Of Rapeseed Oil Is Heated In A Large Pan. Now The Onions Are Fried Until They Are Translucent.

6. Then The Beetroot Is Added Together With Three Tablespoons Of Water.

7. Now The Whole Thing Is Seasoned With A Pinch Of Salt And Pepper And Then Left To Sizzle For Three Minutes Over Medium Heat.

8. Next, The Cream Cheese Is Placed In A Bowl And The Garlic Is Peeled And Pressed Into The Cream Cheese Using A Garlic Press, Stirred And Refined With Salt And Pepper.

9. Now The Chops Are Taken Out Of The Oven And Served With The Cream Cheese Mixture, The Beetroot And The Onions.

10. Finally, the dish is drizzled with a tablespoon of olive oil.

Classic Pasta Pan With Delicious Beans

Ingredients:

- 4 tablespoons of olive oil

- 1 tbsp lemon juice

- 1 tbsp butter

- 110 ml vegetable stock

- 1 pinch of salt and pepper

- 320 g runner beans

- 270 g cherry tomatoes

- 220 g of pasta

- 4 tbsp parmesan

- 2 cloves of garlic

- 30 g basil, savory and chives

Directions:

1. Firstly, the beans are washed, decapitated and cut into bite-sized pieces.
2. Then The Butter Is Melted In A Large Pan, The Beans Are Added And Everything Is Mixed With The Vegetable Stock.
3. Now The Beans Are Sweated Briefly, About 100 Ml Of Water Are Added And Everything Is Simmered For About 15 Minutes With The Pan Closed.
4. In The Meantime You Can Start Washing The Tomatoes And Halving Them And Cooking The Pasta In Salted Water Until Al Dente.
5. Then The Herbs Are Washed And Finely Chopped, The Garlic Cloves Are Peeled And Chopped.
6. Now Herbs, Garlic, Olive Oil, Parmesan And Lemon Juice Are Mixed Together And Finally Refined With Salt And Pepper.

7. Now The Tomatoes Are Added To The Beans And Steamed Again For 5 Minutes.

8. Next, the herb mixture and the cooked noodles are stirred into the beans, mixed well, left to steep and refined again with salt and pepper.

Mediterranean Mashed Potatoes

Ingredients:

- 120 g dried tomatoes

- 60 g pine nuts

- 110 ml of olive oil

- 1 teaspoon lemon juice

- 1 pinch of salt and pepper

- 3 kg of potatoes

- 4 shallots

- 2 cloves of garlic

- 1 bunch of basil

Directions:

1. Firstly, the potatoes are peeled, washed and cooked in salted water.

2. Meanwhile, The Shallots Are Peeled And Finely Diced.

3. Now You Can Peel The Garlic And Cut It Into Thin Slices.

4. Next, The Basil Is Washed, Patted Dry And The Leaves Plucked Off.

5. Finally, The Tomatoes Are Also Finely Diced.

6. Now The Pine Nuts Can Be Roasted Dry In A Pan And Set Aside.

7. Then 2 Tablespoons Of Olive Oil Are Heated, The Shallots And Garlic Are Steamed In Them Until Translucent, Then The Remaining Oil Is Added And Heated.

8. Next, The Potatoes Are Drained, The Oil Poured Over Them And Everything Roughly Mashed.

9. Then The Pine Nuts, Tomatoes And Basil Can Be Mixed In And Everything Can Be Refined With Salt And Pepper.

10. Finally, the dish is rounded off with lemon juice.